75 Successful Weight Loss Tips

OKONGOR NDIFON

DEDICATION

I hereby dedicate this book to all in need of weight Loss, , all over the whole world.

CONTENTS

ACKNOWLEDGMENTS

My acknowledgement goes to all in search of weight Loss.

1 INTRODUCTION

The 75 Successful Weight Loss Tips, are bound to enable you drop that extra fat in your body.

These are expert tips that have been proven to really give successful Weight loss.

Weight loss is a subject that interests a lot of people, with good reason.

Modern life encourages a sedentary, unhealthy lifestyle and offers diet options that can lead to obesity.

Deciding to lose weight is a laudable goal for anyone.

Significant weight loss can spring from humble beginnings; this write up will share a few techniques that may prove highly useful.

Are you finally ready to shed those unwanted pounds, but you aren't sure where to start?

There are so many questions that should be answered when it comes to finding the best way to reach your weight loss goals.

Going through the abundance of information available can become confusing to say the least.

2 75 SUCCESSFUL WEIGHT LOSS TIPS

1. JOIN WEIGHT LOSS SUPPORT GROUP

Consider joining a weight loss support group to help you along your weight loss journey.

This will surround you with people who want to help you with your goals, and give you someone to fall back on when you are tempted to break your diet.

With people surrounding you at all times, you are sure to get motivated to move forward in your weight loss journey.

SOME PLACES TO FIND AND JOIN A WEIGHT LOSS SUPPORT GROUP:

a. Applications(Apps)

Weight loss applications are quite beneficial to those in the journey.

They can assist you in keeping a record of your calorie consumption and physical activity.

Many of these applications also provide social media connections and chat rooms as additional resources.

Examples of weight loss support group Apps to join are:

i. MyFitnessPal

An app called MyFitnessPal, includes a discussion board where you can connect with other users and share advice and success stories.

You can download the app or use the website.

ii. Fitbit App

You can download the app or use their website.

Fitbits are wearable devices that measure your activity level throughout the day.

The devices will help you to track your physical activity.

Fitbit' fitness app also provides robust community features.

When you buy a Fitbit watch, you can connect with other Fitbit users, such as friends and family.

You can take part in challenges with them and even locate a local challenge with strangers.

The app is free.

But to benefit maximally, it offers in-app purchases, such as a monthly $9.99 or a yearly $79.99 subscription.

iii. FatSecret App

The app allows you to log your food intake, monitor your weight, and interact with other people through its community chat feature.

FatSecret allows you to connect with individuals by chatting with them and creating or joining groups.

You can download the app for free.

You can get access to the app's features for a subscription of $6.99 per month or $38.99 for a year

iv. Lose it! App

The app focuses on calories counting and weight tracking.

Lose It! generates your daily calorie needs and a personalized weight loss plan, through an analysis of your weight, age, and health goals.

There are some other good features or highlights of the app, such as challenge, food intake and potion sizes tracker, etc.

The app is free to download.

But to access some premium features, you must pay $9.99 monthly, or sign up for a year for $39.99.

v. WW App

WW or Weight Watchers, is an app that offers various services to

help with weight loss and maintenance.

WW uses a system that helps users stay within their daily calorie allotment to enhance fat loss.

You can partake in WW by attending their in person meetings, which are held in various locations throughout the United States.

You can also participate in their program which is entirely digital through the WW app.

v. Etc

b. Online Forums

You can join online support forums.

Most forums offer a safe place for members to share stories as well as diet and exercise plans.

Members of an online forum can also get motivation.

c. Clinic-Based Support Groups

You can join small weight loss groups at universities or medical centers, if you seek weight loss help from medical professionals.

Medical professionals such as Psychologists, Nutritionists, or other weight loss professionals are those that run these clinic-based support groups.

Joining them can enable you to get individual attention and support, in your weight loss journey.

d. Local Peer Group Support

Getting together with friends locally can be of help in your weight loss journey.

Together with friends can enable you to lose weight faster than doing it alone.

You may learn healthy choices and new habits while you join with friends.

2. DO THIRTY MINUTES OF EXERCISE DAILY.

You can do whatever exercising you feel most comfortable with running, walking, swimming, biking, playing sports, etc.

Since the basic formula for losing weight is taking in less calories than you burn, by exercising each day you'll increase the number of calories you burn daily.

Exercises are good for the body. Try never to miss your daily exercise routine.

HOW TO DO 30 MINUTES OF EXERCISE DAILY

i. Start Small

Start small and gradually Increase the Intensity and duration of your daily exercise and workouts.

Don't start running a marathon race, as a beginner. You may be discouraged or even get injured as you start.

If you are someone new to exercise, begin with walking, jogging, stretching, and jumping or jump rope exercise.

Do any of these simple exercises for 30 minutes each day.

ii. Create and do enjoyable exercises daily

Examples of enjoyable daily exercises are:

- 30 minutes spot matching
- 30 minutes marching forth and back
- 30 minutes dancing
- 30 minutes strolling around your neighborhood
- 30 minutes jogging at home or around your neighborhood
- 30 minutes biking around your neighborhood
- 30 minutes skipping ropes
- 30 minutes jumping at home
- 30 minutes of swimming
- 30 minutes of lifting weights or dumb bells

- 30 minutes of stretching
- 30 minutes of deep breathing and exhaling
- Etc.

iii. Do Different Exercises Daily

Don't do one exercise daily. It may become boring or discouraging.

To prevent boredom, discouragement, and fatigue, you can mix and do indoor and outdoor exercises, activities, and sports, etc.

iii. Create Time to Exercise

Make sure you create a 30 minutes period and avail yourself during this time for exercise.

iv. Make it a Daily Habit

Start exercising and make it a daily habit.

Train yourself daily to exercise, and it shall become a daily habit.

It is said that for someone to imbibe an habit that continues on a daily basis, it takes 21 days.

As such, don't give up too early in trying to form the habit of exercising daily.

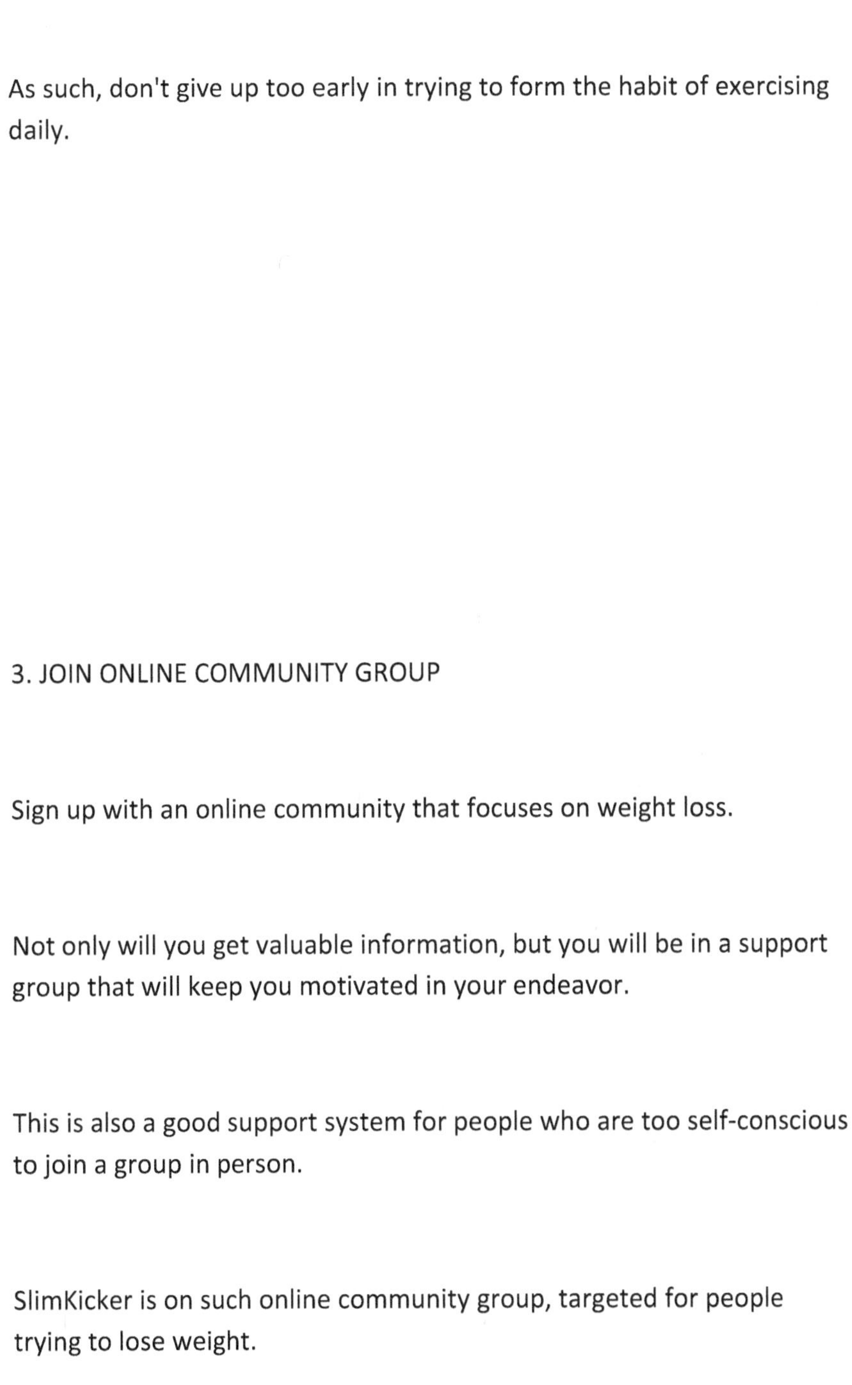

3. JOIN ONLINE COMMUNITY GROUP

Sign up with an online community that focuses on weight loss.

Not only will you get valuable information, but you will be in a support group that will keep you motivated in your endeavor.

This is also a good support system for people who are too self-conscious to join a group in person.

SlimKicker is on such online community group, targeted for people trying to lose weight.

4. GET RIGHT MEAL DAILY

A good way to help you lose weight is to make sure you're getting the right ratio of macro-nutrients for each meal.

Ideally you want to have forty percent of protein, forty percent of carbohydrates, and twenty percent of fat in every meal. Following this basic guideline can produce great results.

To get right meals daily for weight loss, start creating nutrient-dense dishes by

i. filling one-third to one-half of your plate with non-starchy vegetables.

These are low in calories and give plenty of water, fiber, and vitamins and minerals.

ii. Fill a quarter to a third of your plate with protein-rich foods like meat, fish, or legumes, and the rest with nutritious grains, fruit, or starchy vegetables.

These will provide additional protein, vitamins, minerals, and fiber.

iii. Take a splash of healthy fats from foods like avocados, olives, nuts, and seeds.

iv. Eat Right Snacks

If hunger comes between meals, don't eat junk food.

Benefit from eating a right snack to help you get through the time between meals, by eating snacks high in protein and fiber, which are most helpful for weight loss.

The right snacks to eat include, apple slices with peanut butter, vegetables, roasted chickpeas, yogurt, fruits and almonds.

v. Right Foods for Weight Loss

The various right foods to eat during your weight loss journey include:

Yoghurt, soups, beans and legumes, root vegetables, potatoes, chili peppers, lean meat, chicken breast, salmon, white eggs, avocados, cottage cheese, leafy greens, whole grains, nuts, grapefruit, fruits, and vegetables.

5. DON'T DWELL ON PROGRESS

A good way to help you lose weight and be successful with your diet is to not dwell too much about your progress.

Stay busy with work or with your friends and family and try not too much about your weight loss.

Thinking about it too much can cause you to lose motivation because you want to see results right away.

6. REDUCE CARBOHYDRATES INTAKE

Reduce the amount of carbohydrates that you eat throughout the day.

Also do not eat any carbohydrates late in the afternoon or in the evening.

You can increase the amount of good fat and protein that you eat to compensate for your lost calories when you cut out the carbohydrates.

Carbohydrate restriction is a prominent strategy for achieving weight loss.

When you start eating fewer carbs, your body's energy recruitment changes, making you feel different physically and mentally.

Reducing your intake of calorie-dense carbohydrates naturally lowers your daily calorie intake.

This will force your body to burn fat stored around your midsection for energy rather than the sugars it gets from carbohydrates.

The result of fat being used up or burnt that was stored around your midsection, results in weight loss.

What will happen to you when you replace simple carbohydrates with high-fiber foods is that your belly will begin to flatten..

How to Reduce Carbohydrates Intake

i. Keep Yourself Hydrated.

Staying hydrated is one of the most important aspects of overall health.

While you should prevent dehydration if you exercise regularly, even slight dehydration can have a negative impact on your skin and intestinal health.

Proper water is essential for healthy digestion.

 Because low-carb diets might promote constipation, it's critical to drink enough of water every day.

ii. Add Healthy Fats to your meals

As you plan your meal, add, healthy fats for flavor, health advantages, and satiety.

Your body requires fat to function properly, therefore eating a diet rich in healthy fat is critical to your overall health. 9 While

As you avoid eating some saturated fats in your diet, make sure you eat healthy fats.

iii. Eat Whole Grains

Go for whole grains like corn, millet, barley, oats, etc.

iv. Eat Protein Rich Foods

Some good sources of protein include:

Yogurt

Nuts and seeds

Egg

Legumes, beans, and lentils

Soy products

Chicken breast

Fish

Lean meats

v. Eat None Starchy Vegetables

None starchy vegetables include: l greens, peppers, mushrooms, cauliflower, etc.

vi. Avoid Sugary Products

Check processed food products before buying them, in order to avoid hidden sugar they contain.

Make sure you limit the intake of added sugar from beverages.

vii. Eat Quality Potion Size Foods

23

Quality of foods should be preferred over quantity.

viii. Avoid Packaged Snacks

ix. Find Low Carb Snacks

Cutting carbs may help shed pounds.of weight gain.

Processed carbohydrates tend to convert very quickly into sugars while in the body.

If reducing intake of carbohydrates may be difficult, find alternatives to help the matter.

Instead of spending time to look at labels on processed foods, just find alternatives.

7. EAT MORE RAW FOODS

For easier digestion, try including more raw foods in your diet.

Uncooked foods are often easier for your body to break down because their natural enzymes have not been destroyed by the cooking process.

Older people will often have an easier time getting the nutrients they need from raw food.

8. EAT FOODS WITH HEALTHY FATS

A great tip for successful weight loss is to choose foods that have healthy fats like polyunsaturated fat and monounsaturated fat.

These include walnuts, olives, and salmon.

These healthy fats make you full and satisfied for a longer period of time so you will not overeat later in the day.

9. EAT SUGARLESS GUM

When you are trying to lose weight, you should always have some sugarless gum available.

Chewing gum suppresses the appetite. It gives your mouth something to do and the flavor can distract you from cravings.

Mint gums also make your mouth feel clean.

Most people do not want to eat when their mouth feels clean.

10. CARRY FOODS WHEN GOING OUT

A good tip for losing weight is to pack healthy food with you if you're going to be away from home.

A lot of people make the mistake of not packing food with them and they are forced to resort to unhealthy food.

It's best to pack healthy food with you, in case you get hungry.

11. DON'T USE YOUR AUTOMOBILE

When trying to lose weight, using transportation other than automobiles can help.

Walking, bicycling, running, roller blading, and various other physical transportation methods can burn calories.

Calories you've added on through eating are in your body, of which they must be burnt, to lose weight.

12. SNACK VEGETABLES

One great weight loss tip for someone with a busy schedule is to buy bagged, cut up vegetables such as carrots and broccoli.

They are easy to grab as a healthy snack on the go or to put into salads for a meal.

The best part is that they are fresh and have not been frozen or cooked.

13. EAT SOUPS

Eating soup can help you lose weight, especially if you place it in the refrigerator to cool before eating.

Most of the fat from the soup will move to the top of the bowl, allowing you to scoop it out, throw it away and save yourself some calories before you enjoy your meal.

14. TRACK PROGRESS WITH BELT

A great tip to help you lose weight is to track your progress by using your belt.

Scales can be very inaccurate when determining how fit you are, but your belt will let you know if you're losing weight.

If you have to increase a notch or two in your belt, then you are making great progress.

15. CLEAN JUNK FOODS OUT OF YOUR KITCHEN

When you're cleaning your house, why not clean your kitchen of unhealthy foods as well?

Take the time to go through your cupboards, fridge and pantry and toss out all the cookies, chips and other junk food that you have sitting around.

If you allow junk foods to sit around in your kitchen, you may be tempted to consume them. The best thing to do is to get them out of your kitchen.

If they're not there to tempt you, you'll be more likely to eat a healthy diet.

16. ADD SPICES TO MEALS

A good tip that may help you lose weight is to add spices to your meals.

When dieting, a lot of people make the mistake of eating their meals totally bland, without any flavor at all.

You should try adding spices to your meals to keep yourself motivated and interested.

17. EAT SLOWLY

An easy way to restrict your calorie intake is to simply eat more slowly.

Stop, chew, and savor your food. Do not finish a meal within five minutes of sitting down with it.

If you eat too fast, your brain won't be able to send the "full" signal to your stomach in time.

You will end up overeating and most likely gaining weight if you eat too fast.

18. DON'T SKIP MEALS

Make sure you're not skipping meals. Try to eat about three balanced meals each day.

You can still lightly snack on healthy foods.

This helps produce a harmony to your body for top functionality.

19. PLAY BASKETBALL

A great way to motivate yourself to lose weight and get more exercise is to join a team sport.

For example, a game of pickup basketball can burn over a hundred calories in just half an hour.

If you have friends counting on you to show up at an appointed time each weekend, you'll be more likely to go.

20. DRINK FRUIT JUICE INSTEAD OF SODA

Diet sodas may seem like a good idea if you are trying to save on calories while dieting.

People who regularly drink diet soft drinks are more likely to be overweight than their non-diet soda drinking counterparts.

Instead of club soda drinks, go for fruit juice.

21. USE A GYM MACHINE

Which cardio machine burns the most fat?

This comes when you walk into a gym

Your walking into a gym is for you to drop off or shed pounds of weight.

Since weight loss is the goal you have in mind, the following machines are the best to help:

i. ELLIPTICALS

The elliptical is the ideal machine for substantial lower body burn if you want to take your training to another level.

The elliptical is designed to tone your thighs without putting any strain on your knees or ankles like running or jogging would.

This machine is recognized for quickly melting extra fat.

When in the gym to use this machine, make sure you know the best settings for you to use, in order to burn down fat quickly.

A great way to help you lose weight is to hop on the elliptical machine at your gym.

The elliptical machine burns more calories when compared to other machines, such as the stationary bike.

The elliptical machine is also low impact, so you aren't putting that much strain on your joints.

ii. Spinning Bike

I hope you are familiar with the stationary bike, which is designed to seem like a bicycle.

The spinning bike is different from the stationary bike.

A spinning bike will help raise your heart rate and enable you to start losing weight.

 Aside from improving your heart health, a spin cycle is ideal for persons who are prone to injuries, those who want to grow lean muscle, and those who enjoy adjusting their bikes for the most efficient and pleasant ride.

iii. TREADMILL

A treadmill is a terrific way to burn calories when it's too hot outside or you don't have enough space to go for a jog or stroll.

The simple treadmill is a terrific piece of equipment once you've entered your basic information.

A treadmill is a terrific place to start if you're searching for a beginner's weight loss program using gym machines.

You may use this fantastic piece of equipment for everything from long runs to interval training.

This is one of the best ways to lose weight at the gym, whether it's a 60 minute brisk stroll or a 60 second sprint.

You are sure to go with a treadmill, in your weight loss journey.

iv. MACHINE FOR ROWING

While there is no quick remedy for achieving the ideal body, a total body workout can help.

A rowing machine for cardio provides a full body exercise in a matter of minutes.

The machine guarantees a raise in heart rate and burn all throughout your legs, arms, back, and core after the first few pulls!.

You can choose from a variety of modes on this machine.

You must take precautions before and while engaging in rowing, to avoid injury.

Make sure you have the right knowledge on how to use the machine profitably.

Ask the gym attendant for help in using the rowing machine.

22. CONSUME SMALL FOOD

You can consume less calories, and lose more weight, if you take the time to cut up your food.

Portion control is difficult for most people, so take a food that contains a large amount of calories (like chocolate) and cut it into smaller portions.

You can still eat what you like, but by only consuming a small amount of the food, you will not gain as much weight.

23. WEIGHT LOSS IS SLOWLY

If you are desperately in need of losing extra weight, make sure you keep in mind that there is no easy way to lose weight.

There are no magical pills or special machines that are going to make you lose a hundred pounds in a month.

Weight loss is a gradual process.

24. BUY WORKOUT OUTFITS

A great tip that may help you lose weight is to purchase some new workout outfits.

Once you know you've forked out the money for workout outfits, you'll be more inclined to follow through with your weight loss goals because you don't want all that money you spent to be wasted.

25. BUY EXERCISE SHOES

You have to have shoes that fit you well when you are ready to start exercising.

If you are going to be doing extra work outs you need to ensure that you have good shoes.

You don't need to purchase expensive footwear, but make sure that you wear them around a while to ensure comfort and proper fit.

26. EVALUATE HOW HUNGRY

Take a small break during each meal.

Oftentimes, you may be so busy eating that you do not realize that you are actually full.

Make a habit out of stopping midway through a meal. Pause for a minute or so, and try to evaluate how hungry you are.

Use this information to decide whether you need to eat more and how much you want to eat.

27. STOP EATING DONUTS

A great nutritional tip is to say goodbye to donuts.

Donuts are notorious for being very high in fat, and they will sabotage any attempt at trying to lose weight or get fit.

Instead, try spreading some natural peanut butter onto a few slices of whole wheat bread.

28. EAT MORE RAW FOODS

Make raw foods, especially raw vegetables, a cornerstone of any weight-loss diet.

Cooking typically removes vital nutrients and vitamins out of food.

These losses are most evident with vegetables.

Beyond the technical, nutritional benefits, a dieter will likely find that raw, fresh foods taste better than their canned, preserved or cooked, counterparts.

29. BETTER COOK YOUR MEALS

To help you lose weight you can learn to cook for yourself and your family.

There are many people out there that already know how to do this and do it well, yet people often make choices of reheating prepackaged foods.

Learning how to make simple and healthy meals will support your weight loss goals and you will be helping your family eat healthier as well.

30. MAKE EFFORT TO LOSE WEIGHT

It might be difficult to get started and keep to a healthy weight loss strategy.

People frequently lack the ambition to get started or lose motivation to continue.

Fortunately, motivation is something that can be improved.

One important tip for weight loss is this mantra: "plan, prepare, perform, and practice!"

Weight loss doesn't happen by accident, it takes mental effort and deliberate steps in order to achieve the results that you want.

Overcoming inertia and stepping out in action is one of the hardest and most rewarding parts.

Once you start moving forward, the rest will be easier.

How to Make Effort to Lose Weight

i. Set Weight Loss Goals

Clearly outline and write down your weight loss objectives.

For long term success, be sure your motivation comes from within.

ii. Your Weight Loss Goals Must be Realistic

Set realistic weight loss goals to increase feelings of accomplishment and avoid burnout.

Even a small weight loss of some few pounds can have a significant influence on your health.

Rather than setting what is unattainable, which may discourage you, stick to realistic or achievable goals.

To develop realistic goals, consider using SMART goals.

The acronym SMART stands for:

S - Specific

M - Measurable

A - Achievable

R - Realistic

T - Time-based

SMART goals include the following:

a. Daily consumption of five servings of fruits and vegetables

b. 30 minute brisk walk, five days a week, starting next week

c. Daily replacement of soda drinks with fruit juice

d. 60 minutes engagement in the gym next week

iii. Set Plan of Action to Achieve Your Weight Loss Goals

You must do something for you to achieve your weight loss goals.

You have set your realistic weight loss goals and objectives. Do what it will take to help you achieve the goals.

Concentrating solely on the end result can derail your motivation.

The end result of weight loss can feel too far away at times, leaving you feeling overwhelmed, and tired of everything.

Instead, you should action and process goals, or the steps you'll take to get your intended result.

You can for example set an action or process goal of exercising five a week.

As you focus on this action plan or process goal, you are most likely going to achieve your weight loss goal and loss weight.

iv. Pick Eating Plan

Pick an eating plan that you can stick to long term and avoid extreme or quick fix diets.

v. Keep a Weight Loss Journal

Keeping a weight loss journal can help you measure progress, identify triggers and hold yourself accountable.

You must, however, write down everything you consume in order to keep a proper food journal.

This covers all meals, snacks, and the chocolates, including over eating, and emotions.

You can use a website or app as a tool for track or notebook.

31. STOCK UP SPICES

Stock up on cooking spices. Eating healthy while you are trying to lose weight does not mean you only get to eat bland, tasteless foods

Make sure your spice rack is varied and well stocked.

The right spices can make healthy foods taste as delicious as any high calorie alternative.

32. TRY A NEW THING

If you've reached a plateau in your weight loss, try something new.

Shake up your routine a little bit.

Take on a new workout routine, or experiment with different sports and activities.

Don't take the lack of weight loss to heart; sometimes everyone gets stuck at a certain level. The important thing is to keep going.

33. TAKE THE STAIRS

Try taking the stairs if you are serious about losing weight.

You might only burn a few extra calories, but it's still a good idea to take the stairs rather than the elevator when possible.

Weight loss requires dedication and may need many approaches to result in the best results.

Apart from simple dieting, exercise is also needed to burn calories that can accumulate during the day.

Weight loss requires a multifaceted approach to get the best results.

A person trying to lose weight must be committed to changing and acquiring new habits.

34. EAT SALAD

To keep an eye on your weight while dining out, always order the salad instead of other appetizers, which will almost invariably be high in fat.

If the salad contains high-fat items, such as bacon and cheese, ask for those to be omitted.

Ask for the dressing to be served on the side, if they have no fat-free options.

Dressing on the side is usually a good idea in any event, since you can dip your salad in the dressing and control how much of it you eat.

35. COOK YOUR MEALS FROM SCRATCH

To cut back on costs while you cut back your diet, try cooking your meals from scratch.

Cooking homemade meals can be great for weight loss. Many restaurant foods are covered in butter or fattening sauces, and are higher in calories than what you would make at home.

The process of preparing food can also burn a lot of calories.

36. EAT LEGUMES AND BEANS

Legumes and beans of all kinds help greatly when people are trying to lose weight.

Beans have almost no fat, are packed with protein and B vitamins, and satisfy the appetite in a way that extremely low-calorie vegetables don't.

They can provide a healthy and lower-calorie substitute for meat; even for meat lovers.

Legumes lend body and flavor to soups, veggie burgers, ethnic dishes, and many other things.

37. BUY FOODS AND DRINKS IN SMALL AMOUNTS

One really simple tip for weight loss is to buy foods and drinks in smaller packages and portions.

Larger boxes, bags and bottles trigger our brains to grab a bigger handful or to pour more into our bowl or glass.

You are less likely to overeat if the amount of food you start out with is smaller.

38. EAT MORE FRUITS

One simple, yet effective tip for losing weight is to eat more fruits and vegetables.

Fruits and veggies are nutrient dense and fill you up quickly while also providing essential vitamins and minerals.

Replace some of the breads and sweets in your diet with these items and watch the pounds drop off.

Don't just add the fruits and veggies or your diet won't change much and you'll just be adding calories!

39. STAY BUSY

A good way to help you lose weight and be successful with your diet is to not dwell too much about your progress.

Stay busy with work or with your friends and family and try not too much about your weight loss.

Thinking about it too much can cause you to lose motivation because you want to see results right away.

40. COMBINE DIET WITH EXERCISE

When it comes to shedding weight and body fat, combining diet and exercise is more beneficial and effective than using either technique alone.

You cannot lose weight by just following a certain diet.

Healthy eating and exercise habits are essential for weight loss success.

Diet and exercise may not be something you may want to do together.

Dieting simply entails eating nutritious, low-calorie meals. While exercise entails increasing your physical activity.

Although most people focus on diet when trying to lose weight, physical activity is also an important part of any weight-loss plan.

Your body needs energy (calories) to move when you're active, which helps you burn the calories you consume from food.

To lose weight, reduce your calorie intake. However, to maintain a long-term weight loss, include moderate physical activities.

Combining diet and exercise leads to changes that improve body measurements and heart health more than changes in diet or exercise alone.

You must combine eating the right kinds of foods with a strict exercise routine that you are sticking with and following.

A complete lifestyle change is the only way to effectively lose weight and keep it off for good.

While it may be easier to control your calorie intake, regular exercise helps to maintain lean muscle and burn calories.

 Diet and exercise are both vital for weight loss, and combining the two will yield the best results.

Exercise first thing in the morning before eating breakfast. This makes your body burn stored fat rather than the food you ate earlier in the day.

41. SET WEIGHT LOSS GOALS

Set realistic goals when starting a diet.

Like with any other project, if your goals are unattainable, then you have no chance of success.

Regardless of how much you might desire a positive outcome, setting unrealistic goals for yourself is destined for failure.

Each week, try to set a goal to lose at most one pound. Do not try to look too far into the future.

Break it up into attainable weekly goals and focus on reaching each goal.

42. MAKE SURE YOU DRINK WATER

Drinking water is an obvious weight-loss suggestion, but did you know it can also affect your appetite at mealtime?

Next time you're sitting down to dinner, try drinking a large (16-oz or more) glass of cool water before you sit down to eat.

Water can aid weight loss significantly. It is calorie-free, aids in calorie burn, and may even reduce your appetite for food if taken before a meal.

You may find that your stomach has less room for food and that you will eat less.

Weight reduction is dependent on a variety of factors interacting, but there's no doubting that water plays a vital role.

To lose weight and stay healthy, the following reasons show why you must drink water:

i. Water is necessary for nearly all of the body's systems to survive and function properly.

ii.. Water is needed for the metabolic process, to helps our bodies break down fats, in order to lose weight.

iii. Water, makes up 60% of each cell and supporting cell structure of the body.

iv. Water helps digestion by transporting nutrients through our bloodstream.

v. Water is needed for perspiration and respiration which serve to control our interior body temperature.

.

vi.. Water helps to flush waste from our bodies.

vii. Because water has no calories, we can reduce our caloric intake by substituting it for other calorie containing liquids. This helps in weight loss.

43. KEEP AN EYE ON YOUR WEIGHT

To keep an eye on your weight while dining out, always order the salad instead of other appetizers, which will almost invariably be high in fat.

If the salad contains high-fat items, such as bacon and cheese, ask for those to be omitted.

Ask for the dressing to be served on the side, if they have no fat-free options.

Dressing on the side is usually a good idea in any event, since you can dip your salad in the dressing and control how much of it you eat.

44. REDUCE INTAKE OF CALORIES

Weight loss can be achieved through a reduced intake of calories.

If you substitute heavier calorie foods/drinks for nearly identical ones but with less calories, you will find that your weight goes down.

For example, drink diet/light drinks instead of regular drinks and eat frozen yogurt instead of ice cream.

45. DON'T BE IN A HURRY

You need a lot of patience to successfully lose weight.

Crash diets are notorious for being miserable, specifically because they discourage people.

Furthermore, crash diets activate fat retention by fooling the body into starvation mode.

Healthy weight loss should always be gradual. You'll feel better and you'll enjoy long-term health benefits.

46. TAKE FAT BURNING SUPPLEMENTS

A great way to help you lose weight is to invest in a fat burning supplement.

A lot of people make the mistake of relying too much on fat burning supplements.

Instead, you should diet for a while on your own, then utilize a fat burning supplement to help you through the rest of the stretch.

Several natural supplements have been shown to increase fat burning.

Some of the natural supplements for weight loss include:

* Green Tea Extract

* Caffeine

* Soluble Fiber

* Protein Powder

Make sure you consult your doctor before taking them and in any other health impacting changes or medication.

47. ENGAGE IN PHYSICAL ACTIVITIES AND AVOID SEDENTARY LIFE

A practice that will help one lose weight is to replace time spent watching television or movies with time doing physical activities.

Regular physical activity is beneficial to your health, especially if you're attempting to reduce weight or maintain a healthy weight.

More physical activity boosts the number of calories your body uses for energy or for burning fat, during weight loss.

Your calories reduce when you burn calories through physical activity, while you also are reducing the number of calories you eat. This results in weight loss.

The majority of weight loss is due to a reduction in calorie consumption.

However, evidence shows that regular physical activity is the only method to maintain weight loss.

Most importantly, physical activity lowers the risk of cardiovascular disease and diabetes in addition to weight loss.

By exercising in some way as opposed to sitting in a couch or chair will translate into more calories being burned and more healthy activity during time that would have been spent sitting.

Therefore, rather than sitting down endlessly, keep doing little physical activities like going for your daily newspaper instead of sitting and sending for it, fetching water, emptying the trash can, etc, in addition to schedule weekly exercises.

48. TAKE YOGURT

Yogurt is a friend to anyone on a diet.

Select low-fat and plain varieties of yogurt.

Along with a freshly sliced cucumber and some salt and pepper for seasoning, plain yogurt is the perfect ingredient for a crisp, refreshing salad.

You can add fruit to regular yogurt and manage to avoid sugars that are in many yogurts being sold.

Yogurt not only tastes great but is high in calcium.

Best yoghurt for weight loss include:

i. Greek Yogurt

Low fat Greek yogurt has twice the amount of satiating protein as regular yogurt, which might help you feel fuller for longer and regulate your appetite.

This can lead to a reduction in abdominal fat.

Yogurt is also high in calcium, which has been associated to decreased levels of belly fat in studies.

Some best Greek Yogurts are:

* Fage Total 0 % Greek Yogurt

* Light & Fit Two Good Greek Low-Fat Yogurt, Vanilla

* Wallaby Organic No Sugar Added Aussie Greek Yogurt, Peach Hibiscus

* Chobani Non-Fat Plain Greek Yogurt

* Stonyfield Organic Whole Milk Greek Yogurt, Plain

* Maple Hill Creamery Plain Greek Yogurt

ii. YQ Plain Yogurt

iii. Icelandic Provisions, Vanilla Skyr

iv. Siggi's Icelandic Style Strained Non-Fat Vanilla Yogurt

v. Dannon Whole Milk Vanilla Yogurt

49. AVOID HARMFUL DIETS

Do not try diet fads, like weight-loss pills or extreme diet plans.

Many of these methods might be harmful to your overall health in the long run.

In addition, the pounds lost tend to be temporary.

Most people cannot stick to a rigid diet and will, most likely, gain back more than the weight they lost.

50. AVOID FAST FOODS

Order off the kid's menu. Fast food has quite a few calories.

The portions are also much larger than what your body actually needs.

In truth, kid's meals are closer to the correct portion an adult might eat.

Opt for a kid's meal instead of "super sizing" all you food.

51. AVOID FEELING LONELY

Eating out of loneliness is a big problem for many Americans.

Recognizing when you are doing this will help you learn how to break the habit.

You need to find other activities when you feel lonely (chat online, email people, go to a crowded place) and you will find that you will start to lose weight simply by not eating so much.

52. DAILY INCREASE YOUR LEVEL OF PHYSICAL ACTIVITIES

To help you lose weight you should increase your level of physical activity every day.

It does not have to be a large increase since doing any more than you currently do will be burning extra calories as well as building up muscle.

Muscle is more effective at burning calories so even a minimum weight loss is a good start.

53. KEEP A JOURNAL

A good way to lose weight is to start keeping a daily journal of the food you eat.

By keeping a journal of the food you eat, you'll be more inclined to stick with your diet and you can keep track of what foods you like and which ones you don't like.

54. YIELD NOT TO TEMPTATION

Everyone gives in to temptation every now and then.

One way to limit the amount of damage you can do to your diet when you give in to temptation is to limit the amount of fatty temptations around you.

Filling your fridge and pantry with healthier alternatives such as crackers instead of chips, yogurt or fat free pudding instead of ice cream and flavored water instead of soda and you can easily pass on hundreds of calories.

55. AVOID HIGH CALORIES DRINK

Most of us drink coffee or tea. What we put into our hot drinks can be surprisingly caloric.

Starting tomorrow, if you want to help yourself take baby steps to lose weight, dial down the creamer in your coffee.

Better yet, switch to milk. Ramp it down gradually and see if you can get to skim milk (stay away from the artificial fat-free creamer: too fake).

You will find your taste buds adjusting, and with each cup, you'll be taking in significantly fewer calories and animal fats.

Over the course of a typical day of coffee drinking, you will be surprised how many fewer calories you have consumed.

56. AVOID BORING EXERCISE

Although exercise is essential to losing weight it doesn't have to be boring.

Play a sport or do an activity you enjoy for exercise.

If exercise is boring or a chore, you are more likely to stop.

Doing an exercise you like makes you more likely to continue being active and less likely to give up.

57. JOIN ONLINE FORUM

67

Join an on-line forum to help you lose weight.

There are hundreds of people out there who need encouragement and support for weight loss goals.

Search the Internet for groups, find one you are comfortable with and get the on-line support you need to help you through hard times you may face while accomplishing your weight lose goals.

58. EAT RAW FRUITS AND VEGETABLES

Eating raw fruit and vegetables can be a huge help when you are trying to lose weight.

Not only do these foods fill you up and make great snacks between meals, they contain the vitamins and minerals from the plants in their purest form, since they have not been cooked or modified by heat.

59. AVOID EATING LATE AT NIGHT

Avoiding food late at night will help you to lose weight in a hurry.

Late-night eating causes significant weight gain in people because the body does not metabolize food well while it is at rest.

If you can cut out those midnight snacks and late-night dinners, you can begin to shed those pounds quickly.

60. EAT THREE TIMES DAILY

An important part of proper weight loss is to eat at least three times per day.

Skipping meals only lowers your metabolism and therefore causes you to gain weight, or lose it more slowly.

Make sure that you eat a healthy breakfast within 30 minutes of getting up in the morning and then another meal every 3-4 hours after that.

61. HAVE EARLY WORKOUTS

In an effective weight-loss exercise routine, it can be very helpful to schedule your workouts as early in the day as you can.

Exercising first thing in the morning provides you with increased energy levels throughout the day.

It also helps your mood, because all day long you can be proud of the fact that you already got your workout done.

62. NEVER MIND YOUR SCALE.

Ignore what your scale says.

A lot of people find themselves easily discouraged when their scale does not indicate that they are making immediate progress.

If you are exercising and dieting properly, just ignore the scale entirely.

Keep up what you are doing. It might take a little while, but eventually you will begin to see results.

63. WALK SOMETIMES

When you arrive at work, park your car as far away from the entrance door as possible.

The calories burned by this extra walking every work day can really add up and help you lose weight faster.

If you use public transport, get off the train or bus a stop before your destination and walk the extra distance.

65. REDUCE CARBOHYDRATES INTAKE

Reduce the amount of carbohydrates that you eat throughout the day.

Also do not eat any carbohydrates late in the afternoon or in the evening.

You can increase the amount of good fat and protein that you eat to compensate for your lost calories when you cut out the carbohydrates.

66. GET RID OF SOME CLOTHES

Get rid of clothes that do not fit you anymore.

Motivate yourself to keep the weight off by only buying clothes that fit your body now.

Remove any clothes that are now too large for you from your wardrobe.

You can donate them to charity or sell them for a tidy sum.

67. DON'T WEIGH DAILY

A key tip for anyone embarking on a weight loss program is to shift focus away from the number on the scale.

Weighing oneself on a daily basis can seriously undermine weight loss efforts, because the normal fluctuations that will surely register on the scale can have a devastating impact on motivation and morale.

A better strategy is concentrate on positive changes in body shape and muscle tone, rather than on actual weight in pounds.

68. SWITCH TO DIET

Switch to diet from soda to lose weight.

You would probably be shocked to know how many calories a day you are getting just from your sugared sodas.

If you trade one super-sized soda for a no-calorie diet soda instead, you can cut 400-500 calories. Multiply that over several drinks a month, or a week, and you can see how quickly that adds up.

69. AVOID SUGARY DRINKS

When you are trying to lose weight, consider cutting out sugary drinks such as soda, iced drinks have almost no nutritional value in them and are simply empty calories.

Instead, drink more water. Water contains no calories and has many benefits for your body.

70. EAT ENOUGH DAILY CALORIES

In order to lose weight properly, be sure to eat enough calories per day.

Starvation diets of sorts are extremely bad for your body for many reasons.

One such reason is that without food intake, your body will slow down its metabolism and attempt to hang onto the energy that you have already stored in the form of fat.

This type of "diet" also leads to binge eating and a sure way to gain the weight back quickly once you do resume normal eating.

71. EAT MORE NUTS

Eat more nuts when you are trying to lose weight.

Nuts are a great snack food and can be used in place of meat in salads and stir-fries.

There are a wide variety of nuts, so that you won't get bored of eating them.

You can even soak nuts in water before you eat them for a different texture.

72. DO DIFFERENT EXERCISE

If you find yourself hitting a plateau in your weight loss or fitness goals, try mixing up your exercise routine a bit once in a while.

Work different muscles and areas of your body and you may be able to burn off more of the fat that your previous routine wasn't targeting.

75

73. AVOID ALCOHOL INTAKE

Keep your alcohol intake to a zero level, especially in your diet and exercise program, for maximum results.

Alcohol inhibits and lowers your metabolism, as well as being high in calorie content. These calories have no nutritional value and are known as empty calories.

74. ENGAGE IN ACTIVITY

When you feel stressed, engage in an activity instead of relying on food as a source of comfort.

Comfort food cannot take away your stress, but it can work against you later when you feel guilty about overeating and gaining those pounds.

If you go out for a walk instead, it will curb your desire to seek comfort food, and you will work off calories at the same time.

75. AVOID OVEREATING AND HIGH CALORIES

Make sure you control your hunger with meals that satisfy to avoid overeating.

Overeating can sabotage an entire diet that day.

You generally know you have reached this point because you start to feel uncomfortable and have a "stuffed" feeling in your stomach.

When your body is telling you to stop, you need to stop eating.

One vital tip for successful weight loss is to avoid over eating and drinks with high amounts of calories.

Even though some fruit drinks can be good for you, some have high amounts of sugar and calories.

The best thing you can drink is water. Most of your body is composed of water.

 Therefore, it makes sense that your body needs water, in order to operate effectively and efficiently.

As a bonus tip for successful weight loss, you must maintain a good quality sleep.

You must sleep sufficient enough on a daily basis, to enhance weight loss.

Experts say, that adults who aren't sleeping enough or getting poor quality sleep after weight loss appear less successful at maintaining weight loss than those with sufficient sleep.

There's a lot of evidence that obtaining less than the recommended amount of sleep per night, which is about 8 hours, will slow down your metabolism.

This slow down of metabolism, will result in weight gain instead of weight loss.

Chronic sleep deprivation has been linked to changes in appetite hormones, and some studies have found a link between poor eating choices and decreased sleep.

Try to maintain a 8 hours sleep, sufficient enough to aid your weight loss journey.

7 CONCLUSION

Looking your best is what everyone wants.

If you feel you'll look better as a slimmer person, losing weight is a necessity.

People want to lose weight for a variety of reasons, and many fall prey to fad diets that promise quick results.

While there are strategies to speed up your weight reduction, it's crucial to remember that losing weight too quickly can be injurious to your health..

This weight loss book has provided safe, successful, and long term weight loss, to help you lose weight.

Get to know that like so many other aspects of life, it is more about the process, journey, and destination, than a scale based approach and a fixed deadline.

These 75 Successful Weight Loss Tips have worked for many others, and they will work for you, if you keep at it.

Commit to losing weight and look your best soon.

To your success in weight loss.

ABOUT THE AUTHOR

I am Okongor Ndifon. I love to write books related to everyday challenges and issues that people face and endeavor to give genuine solutions.